The Master Cleanser

To further expand your knowledge
and eliminate your limitations.
Stanley Burroughs has perfected Color Therapy
and The Vita Flex control system in a book
entitled "Healing For The Age Of Enlightenment"

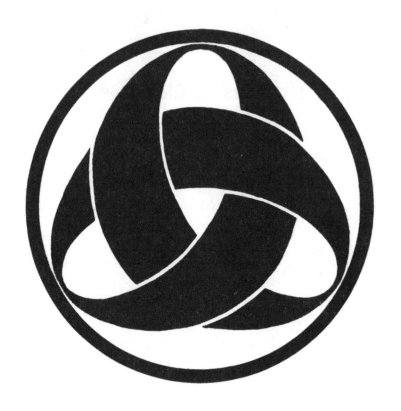

When you learn to know my ways, my ways
will be your ways, in tune with the universal
principals of the fullness of living in
harmony with the universal mind.

The Universal One

Perhaps it is a good thing that medicine and nature never got together — nature could have very easily suffered the many dangerous side effects.

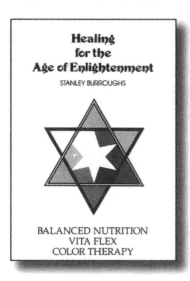

Healing
for the
Age of Enlightenment
STANLEY BURROUGHS

BALANCED NUTRITION
VITA FLEX
COLOR THERAPY

Discover the complete works of Stanley Burrough:

Developed through a lifetime of practice and teaching. His complete system is second to none when properly utilized to promote health & well being.

The Master Cleanser

The most effective cleansing program available, it is simple and inexpensive and can be used by anyone. The results speak for themselves.

Vita-Flex

A pressure point therapy that accesses the more than 5,000 reflex points that are on the body. This technique induces the body to heal itself when one part of the body is activated. Energy then follows meridians to the appropriate reflexive area of the body.

Color Therapy

Color Therapy is the shining of specific colors or frequencies of light on the body to create balance. learn how this ancient therapy can be used as an adjunct to any therapy you may be using.

For Your Information

Healing for the Age of Enlightenment
$13.00

The Master Cleanser
$6.50

To order contact:
faponte@sbcglobal.net

ISBN 0-9639262-0-9

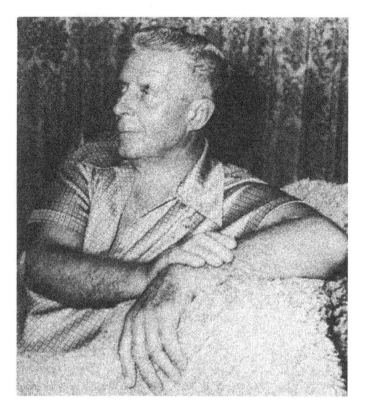

Stanley Burroughs

To bring you hope
To bring you knowledge
To bring you the truth

I present this book so that you can help yourself and others. Make the most of this work and know that it is the finest of knowledge in healing.

"Let no man refuse to listen and be healed lest he bring misery, pain and suffering to those who look and depend on him for help and guidance."

The Blessing

Asking God to bless the food before a meal has been an accepted ritual handed down from generation to generation. It has been thought by some to promote better nutrition and healing by raising the vibration of the food.

Better that we ask God to bless our proper selection of more complete foods as we go shopping for that which will advance our physical and our spiritual needs.

Ask Him to bless the preparation of the food, and for temperance in eating, so as to enable our bodies to receive the utmost of value from what God has so abundantly supplied for our daily use.

Ask Him to bless the animal, fish, or fowl we did NOT kill that we may better sustain our lives with the finer qualities of live fresh fruit, vegetables, and seeds.

Better to ask God to give us KNOWLEDGE to keep our bodies strong and healthy so we have no need to ask Him to heal a sick and ailing body that we produced ourselves by not originally obeying His simple laws.

Blame not God for the many illnesses and diseases you have created (they are not "Acts of God"!). Better that you ask God for His blessings and forgiveness — and to give strength and wisdom to properly apply the knowledge of His simple laws.

CHAPTER I:

The Master Cleanser

For the novice and the advanced student alike, cleansing is basic for the elimination of every kind of disease. The purpose of this book is to simplify the cause and the correction of all disorders, regardless of the name or names. As we eliminate and correct one disease, we correct them all, for every disease is corrected by the same process of cleansing and building positive good health.

Man's mastery of disease will only be final when ignorance and fear are overcome by proper observance of all laws pertaining to the creation of bones, flesh and blood.

Through eons past and on even into the present, man has been held and still remains in bondage of misery and suffering while witchcraft and quackery, whether licensed or not, have run the gamut of the healing field of mis-information.

At last the basic cause of disease is no longer a mystery. The basic cause is the habits of improper diet, inadequate exercise, negative mental attitudes, and lack of spiritual attunement which combine to produce toxic conditions and malfunction of our bodies. The elimination of the cause of illness is the obvious and only way to healing and health. The elimination of the habits that cause illness is done through the positive approach of developing proper habits that cause health combined with corrective techniques that remove the ill effects of our former incorrect ways.

A group of simple and automatic laws of the master plan, for creative living, has given the sufferer his answer and release from his various forms of disease.

These laws pertaining to the construction and reconstruction of a more perfect body are unlimited within the universal plan for man.

Though we have seen and felt the action of these laws as they automatically create and recreate, in our many phases of living, we have discovered and used them knowingly, only in limited amounts.

As we work knowlingly with these laws we find a very simple answer to our many aches, pains and disorders.

To most of us these laws have been replaced with the laws of "Kill of Cure" with the many devastating practices and miracle poisons.

These truths are self evident as we look into the history of our diseases and see our failures in our constant search for release. If these records are not enough then let him go on and on with his never ending aches and pains until his sufferings have finally created a desire for knowing these many truths.

When we finally become sick of being sick, then we are ready to learn the truth and the truth shall set us free. This diet will prove that no one needs to live with his diseases. Lifetime freedom from disease can become a reality.

To be complete, a healing system must be able to cover the entire field of human experiences — physically, mentally and spiritually.

Any system which denies any part of this trinity fails in its attempt to heal to the same extent to which it denies any part or parts.

We realize that many psychological, mental and social stresses can and do cause tensions which can aggravate our problems but they do not cause our conditions. However, the above tensions can and do encourage us to eat to excess — both good and bad foods — which in turn creates our large variety of diseases.

The following program has been tested and approved since 1940 in all sections of the world as the most successful of any diet of its type. Nothing can compare with its positive approach toward perfection in the cleansing and healing field. Nothing can compare with its rapidity and completeness. It is superior in every way as a reducing and body conditioning diet.

As the orginator of this superior diet, I humbly and yet proudly offer it to you, confident that you will receive vigorous good health from its use.

Many of the principles that are presented in this book may be completely contrary to everything you have believed and studied. Regardless of whether you believe them or not, it does not alter the fact that they may be true. Before you attempt to argue or deny these facts, test them as given to you and use them until you have proven them either right or wrong. Every statement and bit of information given is the accumulation

2

of years of experience, research, and results-therefore given as facts. Make these tests and be completely satisfied that you, too, can experience the same results. At no point will any attempt be made to confuse you with theories that cannot be proven or that will not prove themselves to be right. There is no desire to give you complications, or words that have little meaning, or "double talk" without clarity. Simplicity and accuracy will be the theme through the entire book.

This system accepts no limitations as to the ability of the body to heal itself.

"A Letter From One Who Tried it All"
Missing a meal won't hurt!
By Herman Schneider

Since the days of Jesus Christ, who fasted for 40 days, men and women have abstained from food for many reasons; for health, for political ends, and for spiritual enlightenment.

However, the average person, not familiar with fasting, believes he will certainly die if he misses a meal. When you hear of a person dying after being lost in the woods or at sea for two or three days. It was not lack of food that caused his death, but it was panic and fear that killed him. Most people in fairly good health can go for many days without food but the body must have water, although there is a fast called·"the dry fast" which employs dry bread but no liquid. However, this type of fast cannot be endured for too long a period.

There is general disagreement in the health field on the best way to detoxify the body. The Hygienists, who are mostly followers of Dr. Herbert Shelton, the very capable exponent of fasting, using only distilled water, and enemas are taboo. Dr. Shelton and other Hygienist doctors have fasted thousands of people, many regaining their health, as a result of the fast. Of course, after the fast, it was necessary for them to follow a healthful way of life. The Hygienists are strict vegetarians with the emphasis on raw foods and proper combinations.

Dr. Walker and Dr. Airola advocate fruit and vegetable juice if fasting is needed. In Europe, naturopaths use the vegetable broth and vegetable juice fast rather than the water fast. The above doctors also employ colonics and enemas, these being vital for the success of the program. The purpose, in their opinion, is to rid the body of the toxins loosened by the cleanse.

Thirteen years ago, I had extremely high blood pressure. I didn't feel too well, so I went to the doctor. He gulped as he said to me, "your blood pressure in 200 over 120."

He told me that he would start me on medication, but I did not think that drugs were the answer for me, so I asked him, "How long do I have to stay on drugs?" He replied, "Your hypertension will get progressively worse, so you will have to stay on the medicine forever." He continued, "in thirty years of practice, I have had only tow patients able to discontinue the medicine."

I was not pleased with his answer, so I said, "You are looking at your third patient who will get off the medicine."

He looked at me and shrugged his shoulders as if to say, "He is insane." He said, "I have hundreds of patients on medication for high blood pressure, and you are the only one who makes a fuss."

I took one drug for a week, but it made me dizzy, so he changed the medicine. He gave me one drug for high blood pressure and another for nerves, which slowed me down; then another drug to pep me up from the drug that was slowing me down.

CHANGED PROGRAM

I decided this program was not for me, so I headed for Dr. Shelton's in San Antonio, Texas. They took all my drugs and threw them away and put me to bed to start my fast. I never dreamt I would go without food so long, but my fast lasted for 21 days on just distilled water.

It is during the fast that conditions a person may have, but is not yet aware of, show up, as the body begins throwing off the poisons. The man fasting in the next room passed gallstones on his 24th day. He never know he had gallstones before his fast. He really suffered until he passed his stones. after long years of study in natural healing and herbology, I now know he could have gotten rid of the gallstones in a much more pleasant way, using apple juice, olive oil and lemon juice.

I, myself, had mild reactions outside of extreme weakness. My biggest problem was painful cramps caused by gas in the intestines. I also has some bleeding as the bowel tried to empty itself with no bulk ingested to help it move.

My fasting problems would have been much less had they given me an enema, but the Hygienists do not believe in enemas, laxatives or herbs. They say nature must take its course.

The faster is kept in bed most of the time, using one's energy to detoxify.

During the 21 days of fasting, I lost 21 pounds, which I gradually gained back during the rebuilding process, which should equal the fasting time. So I had to stay off of my job for 42 days.

The fast was not pleasant, although you lose your desire for food after the third day. but the results were very pleasant and made it worthwhile; my blood pressure was now 120 over 80 which is perfect.

Since this fast, thirteen years ago, I have fasted many times on vegetable juices and used colonics as advocated by Dr. Walker. The fasts were of short duration, lasting from two to five days.

About a year ago, I went to a chiropractor for an adjustment. We talked for a while and he told me he was on a book called the "Master Cleanser" by Stanley Burroughs, a natural healer for some forty or more years.

The cleanse starts with a herbal laxative tea both morning and evening. If this is not sufficient to clean out the intestinal tract, he advises a salt water wash. These steps are necessary to remove the toxins loosened by the lemon juice cleanse.

I was then to drink between six and twelve glasses of lemonade, which consisted of lemon and maple syrup in proper proportions, with a small amount of cayenne added to wash out the mucus loosened by the cleanse.

I stayed on the *"Master Cleanse"* for 12 days, during which I exercised, jogged, worked, and felt stronger each day, as the cleanse proceeded. I gradually tapered off the cleanse, with juices and broth, for three more days. During the entire time I was never hungry.

The most important part of the cleanse or any fast is knowing how to come off of the fast, allowing the body to gradually adjust itself to handling solid food again. Improper procedures can cause illness and even death.

Since my weight was stabilized when I started the cleanse, I only lost about four pounds in twelve days. People who are overweight will loose much more.

Mr. Burroughs' program calls for a vegetarian diet, so this part of the program was easy for me to accept because I have been a vegetarian for years, using mostly raw foods.

I go on this cleanse two or three times a year. I just read in Linda Clark's book that she has used this cleanse for years.

Mr. Burroughs says that it is perfectly safe to stay on the *"Master Cleanser"* even up to 40 days, as the lemon, maple syrup and cayenne pepper act as both a cleanser and a body builder.

From my viewpoint, the Burroughs cleanse gave me the best results, allowing me to be active and energetic through the entire period.

I haven't been back to the medical doctors, but my blood pressure is still normal after all these years.

A Word About "Epidemics" and "Germ-Caused" Diseases

Throughout the history of man, there have been constant epidemics of many diseases. Little has been known or understood as to why these things happen. (In earlier times they were thought variously to be the work of the devil, punishment from God, or poisoning of the water supply by an enemy). In recent times it has been believed that these many diseases are contagious and that germs have spread them. This belief has created a monster as the medical field has steadily found stronger and more potent drugs, poisons, and antibiotics in their constant effort to destroy what they believe to be the cause. A large variety of vaccines and antitoxins have been developed because of the belief in a large variety of bacteria and viruses.

Always the belief is that we must kill these forms of life in order to keep us free from disease. Yet, in spite of massive research, manufacturing, and wide use of these items, mankind still goes on suffering from an ever-increasing variety of disease and disorders with no let up in sight.

Disease, old age, and death are the result of accumulated poisons and congestions throughout the entire body. These toxins become crystallized and hardened, settling around the joints, in the muscles, and throughout the billions of cells all over the body.

It is presumed by orthodox medicine that we have a perfectly healthy body until something, such as germs or viruses, comes along to destroy it, whereas actually the building material for the organs and cells is defective and thus they are inferior or diseased.

Lumps and growths are formed all over the body as storage spots for unusable and accumulated waste products, especially in the lymphatic glands. These accumulations depress and deteriorate in varied degrees, causing degeneration and decay. The liver, spleen, colon, stomach, heart, and our other organs, glands, and cells come in for their share of accumulations, thus impairing their natural action. These growths and lumps appear to us as forms of fungi. Their spread and growth is dependent on the unusuable waste material throughout the body. As the deterioration continues, our growths increase in size to take care of the situation. Fungi absorb the poisons and try to take the inferior material from the organs. This is a part of Nature's plan to rid the body of our diseases. When we stop feeding this fungi and cleanse our system, we stop their development and spread; then they dissolve or break up and pass from the body. They will not feed on healthy tissue. There is a simple set of laws which explains this action. Nature never produces anything it does not need and it never keeps anything it does not use. All unused material or waste is broken down by bacteria action into a form that can be used over again or eliminated from the body. All weak and deficient cells, caused from improper nutrition will also be broken down and eliminated from the body.

We spend a good portion of our lives accumulating these diseases and we spend the rest of our lives attempting to get rid of them — or die in the effort!

The incorrect understanding of the above truths has led uncivilized and civilized nations alike to search for some magic "cure" in all kinds of charms, witchcraft, and unlimited kinds of obnoxious poisons and drugs. In general, they are worse than useless because they cannot possibly eliminate the cause of any disease. They can only add more misery and suffering and shorten one's life still further. It has been reported in many books and magazine articles that many new diseases and disorders have been created by orthodox and hospital methods.

As we continue to search for more and more magic "cures" we become more and more involved with complicated varieties of disease. A simple understanding and action has always proved to be the best to eliminate our negative actions and reactions.

Germs and viruses do not and cannot cause any of our diseases, so we have no need for finding various kinds of poisons to destroy them. **In fact, man will never find a poison or group of poisons strong enough to destroy all the billions upon billions of these germs without destroying himself at the same time.**

These germs are our friends, there are no bad ones, and if given a chance will break up and consume these large amounts of waste matter and assist us in eliminating them from the body. These germs and viruses exist in excess only when we provide a breeding ground in which they can multiply. Germs and viruses are in the body to help break down waste material and can do no harm to healthy tissues.

Do you think that if an insignificant, microscopic microbe can appear and make you sick when you were well and strong, that you have any possibility of getting strong enough to throw them off at any time thereafter? Do you think that any destructive poisons can make it possible for you to get well any faster?

All diseases, regardless of their names, come within this understanding as only varied expressions of the one disease of **toxemia.**

As noted earlier, we are constantly told that the medical researchers are about to make a big breakthrough and finally conquer all our diseases. This breakthrough will never happen until their false approach to science is replaced by the natural science of the secret of life energy and its creative action within us. Through an open-minded approach to the truth about the life force or energy, we can know the underlying facts behind epidemics and eliminate their cause.

Basically, all of our diseases are created by ourselves because we have never taken the time to discover the true foods meant for man's use. We can create healthy bodies by using the right foods and eliminating highly toxic and mucus-forming foods.

As you learn more about nutrition you will become aware of the many foods that cause excess mucus in our bodies and then realize that this condition becomes the breeding ground for all kinds of germs.

We know that throughout nature everything moves in cycles, constantly changing, constantly cleaning out the old and building the new. Consequently, as a person reaches the "point of no return," a point where his accumulations have reached the limit of what the body can tolerate, then a rapid change takes place or he dies. The cycle has come to the point where a good house cleaning must be started, and one of nature's most effective methods is to start loosening and eliminating these poisons with bacteria action. As this action progresses, we become sick and feverish; large amounts of mucus are eliminated; diarrhea increases the discharge of waste material; and all of our resources go into action to clean us out as fast as possible to prevent these poisons from killing us. When this happens do not panic and resort to the unnatural action of drugs and antibiotics which can only defeat natures laws. The drugs stop the natural changes by suppressing the cleansing action and stores the poisons in the body to cause future problems.

If we know these danger signals and engage our abilities in their maximum effort, we can survive the ordeal and live a normal life until further accumulations trigger another life change. However, the logical procedure is **to prevent these accumulations from forming in the first place** — then we have no need for the discomfort of the severe cleansing process.

As the above conditons happen to more and more people at the same time an "epidemic" is set in motion. Very often an epidemic occurs after holiday feasting. Even the very best of foods in excess can create problems. If only a sufficient amount of good food is consumed, a severe cleansing-illness-will not be required as the normal operation of the body will then be adequate.

Deficiencies do exist, primarily because of improper diet and improper assimilation. These deficiencies also produce toxins because of the deterioration of the cells. So we still have only one disease, and with one simple process we can eliminate all so-called diseases of whatever name. As we expel the disease-producing toxins from our bodies, we must also restore the deficiencies. Thus, a cleansing diet **must also include proper material for building as the waste material is eliminated.**

There is still one more factor involved to make the total process completely understandable. Since germs do not cause our disorders, there must be another logical reason for the triggering of an epidemic. This is a matter of simple "vibration." The better the physical and mental condition a person is in, the higher becomes his vibration, but as he steadily becomes clogged with more and more waste matter, his vibration goes constantly downward until he is ready and in need of a change. If he then comes in contact with one or more who have already started the cleansing process, he picks up the vibration of change and all his functions are triggered into the same action. This can happen to any size group of people in similar condition, and then an epidemic is on its way. The person with a toxic free body and undisturbed mind is the one unaffected by the epidemic.

9

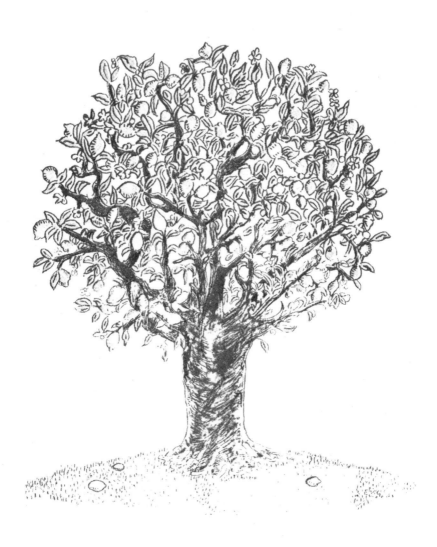

Our Family Tree
Lemons and Limes

The Origin of the Lemonade Diet

The lemonade diet, about to be described, has successfully and consistently demonstrated its eliminative and building ability.

Lemons and limes are the richest source of minerals and vitamins of any food or foods known to man, and they are available the year round. Thus the diet may be used successfully any month of the year and virtually any place on earth. Its universal appeal and availability make it pleasant and easy to use.

The lemonade diet first proved itself in the healing of stomach ulcers over forty years ago. Permission was given by Bob Norman to share this incident of my first experience with the diet.

One day, shortly prior to my first meeting with Bob, I was inspired to write this diet in complete form as a means to give relief and to heal stomach ulcers in ten days. I rapidly wrote it down in detail and waited for a test case — which always seemed to come when it was needed.

Bob Norman had suffered with his ulcer for nearly three years. During this time he had tried everything then known to get help, but nothing in the way of medicine or treatment gave anything but momentary relief. He had to eat something every two hours or he was in extreme pain. For the preceding three months he had been living on little other than goats milk. His doctor wanted to operate but he refused to have it done. He figured anything would be better than that. He told me I was the last person he would go to. If I couldn't help him, he would just go home and die, as life was hardly worth living in this condition.

An explanation of the cause of an ulcer is necessary at this point. There is a sodium coating covering the entire inside wall of the stomach which, if it remains intact, will prevent the digestive juices from digesting the stomach itself. However, when any form of flesh food enters the stomach, the meat attracts the sodium in the same way as the walls of the stomach. Some of the sodium is drawn from the walls and gathers around the meat, thus preventing the digestion of the meat in the stomach and at the same time depleting the sodium on the walls of the stomach.

As one continues to eat meat and a deficiency of sodium in the diet occurs, the sodium lining is not being replaced on the walls of the stomach. The digestive juices then start digesting the stomach, producing what we call an ulcer. When this occurs, all orthodox methods to heal the ulcer fail completely.

11

Sometimes the meat can remain in the stomach for two or more hours and begin to ferment and spoil. To be broken down and digested it must pass on into the small intestine. All forms of meat take longer to digest than do fruit and vegetables. Chicken and other fowl take the longest of all. Just because meat is already a form of flesh, it does not follow that it is readily usable by our bodies. In fact, just the reverse is true.

When one considers that flesh foods of all kinds are extremely toxic, it becomes apparent that they are an extremely undesireable form of nourishment. In the eating of meat, one must take into account all of our eliminative organs. They are made primarily to take care of **our own wastes.** When we add animal flesh, containing the wastes of its cells (or drugs and other unusable materials), extra work is required of these organs and various forms of trouble will eventually develop.

Remember that all solid food must be broken down into a liquid form to be carried by the blood before it can nourish the body. Flesh foods of all kinds (including fish) take much longer to reach this state and are less useful to the body than fruit, vegetables, and seeds.

Back to our story. After all of Bob's explanation, I asked him if he would like to have his ulcer healed in ten days. He answered "Yes" so I handed him the paper with the diet on it. He read it over carefully and handed it back with the explanation that he could never do that as all expert advice for three years had told him to never use citrus, and this was nothing but lemonade.

Since orthodox methods had failed completely to heal his ulcer, I reasoned that their advice could be wrong. And since the lemonade diet was **contrary** to the accepted practices (which had failed), logic told me that it might do the healing. I knew it could do no harm and was confident only good could come from it.

I explained to Bob that if all of this expert advice was correct, his ulcer would have been healed three years ago! It was just possible that the very thing he was told not to use might be the one thing he needed. He thought it over and decided, "All right, I'll try it . . . even if it kills me!" He was assured that this would not happen.

After five days of the diet Bob called me. Even though he had no pain from the beginning, he was afraid that suddenly all the old pain would return and he would be miserable again. Formerly he had to eat something every two hours or he would be in pain, and the previous day he had gone eight hours without food or drink — with no pain, yet he was still apprehensive. I assured him that since he had no pain for five days, he would be all right and to continue for the full ten days.

On the eleventh day he was examined by his doctor and the ulcer had been completely healed. Needless to say, his doctor was most amazed because he had given Bob a complete examination, including X-ray, prior to the diet and had recommended an immediate operation because he would not have long to live otherwise.

Many other cases of ulcers followed with the same constant results in only ten days. Numerous other disorders were also corrected during the ten day period, in person after person.

Is the Lemonade Diet Also a Reducing Diet?

As a reducing diet it is superior in every way to any other system because it dissolves and eliminates all types of fatty tissue. Fat melts away at the rate of about two pounds a day for most persons — and without any harmful side effects.

All mucus diseases such as colds, flu, asthma, hay fever, sinus and bronchial troubles are rapidly dissolved and eliminated from the body, leaving the user free from the varied allergies which cause difficult breathing and clogging of the sinus cavities. Allergies exist as a result of an accumulation of these toxins and they vanish as we cleanse our body. People who are over-weight often experience these difficulties, and the more they continue to eat the toxic fat-producing foods which cause their obesity, the more their other ailments multiply.

Mucus disorders are brought about by the eating or drinking of mucus-forming foods. In other words, if you have these diseases, **you ate them!** As we stop feeding our family mucus-forming foods, we can eliminate their mucus and allergy diseases for the rest of their lives.

The types of disease which are a result of calcium deposits in the joints, muscles, cells and glands are readily dissolved and removed from the body. Cholesterol deposits in the arteries and veins also respond to the magic cleansing power of the lemonade diet.

All skin disorders also disappear as the rest of the body is cleansed. Boils, abscesses, carbuncles, and pimples all come under this category. These conditions are, again, Nature's effort to eliminate poisons quickly from the body.

All types of infections are the result of these vast accumulations of poisons being dissolved and burned or oxidized to produce further cleansing of the body. Therefore, rapid elimination of the toxins relieves the need for infectious fevers of all kinds. Infections are not "caught," they are created by Nature to assist in burning our surplus wastes.

Yes, the lemonade diet is a reducing diet, **but much more.** Just as many other disorders also cleared up at the same time when it was used to heal ulcers, when it is used as a reducing diet other ailments are also corrected in the process.

People build strong, healthy bodies from the correct foods or they build diseased bodies from incorrect foods. When disease does become necessary, the lemonade diet will prove its superior cleansing and building ability.

NOTE

THE FOLLOWING DIET IS GIVEN SOLELY AS
A SUGGESTION; ANYONE WHO FOLLOWS IT
DOES SO VOLUNTARILY. SINCE EACH PER-
SON, NATURALLY, REACTS DIFFERENTLY,
EACH INDIVIDUAL MUST USE HIS OWN
JUDGMENT AS TO ITS USE.

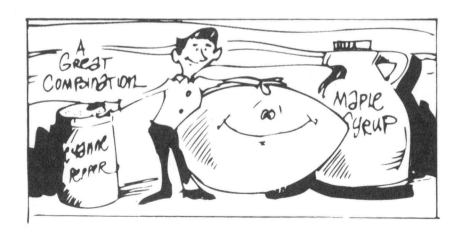

CHAPTER II:

The Master Cleanser
or
The Lemonade Diet

Purpose

To dissolve and eliminate toxins and congestion that have formed in any part of the body.

To cleanse the kidneys and the digestive system.

To purify the glands and cells throughout the entire body.

To eliminate all unusable waste and hardened material in the joints and muscles.

To relieve pressure and irritation in the nerves, arteries, and blood vessels.

To build a healthy blood stream.

To keep youth and elasticity regardless of our years.

When to Use It

When sickness has developed — for all acute and chronic conditions.

When the digestive system needs a rest and a cleansing.

When overweight has become a problem.

When better assimilation and building of body tissue is needed.

And How Often?

Follow the diet for a minimum of 10 days or more — up to 40 days and beyond may be safely followed for extremely serious cases. The diet has all the nutrition needed during this time. Three to four times a year will do wonders for keeping the body in a normal healthy conditions. The diet may be undertaken more frequently for serious conditions.

How to Make It

2 Tbsp lemon or lime juice (approx. 1/2 lemon)
2 Tbsp genuine maple syrup (not maple flavored sugar syrup)
1/10 Tsp cayenne pepper (red pepper) or to taste
Water, medium hot (spring or purified water)

Combine the juice, maple syrup, and cayenne pepper in a 10 oz. glass and fill with medium hot water. (Cold water may be used if preferred.)

Use fresh lemons or limes only, never canned lemon or lime juice nor frozen lemonade or frozen juice. Use organic lemons when possible.

The maple syrup is a balanced form of positive and negative sugars and must be used, not some "substitute". There are four U.S.D.A. approved grades of maple syrup. The early sap runs generally produce the lighter grades - Grade A Light Amber and Grade A Medium Amber, which were formerly known simply as Grade A. These lighter grades are mild in taste, sweet and with less mineral content than the darker grades. The mid-season runs generally yield mostly Grade A Dark Amber, formerly known as Grade B. Dark Amber has more mineral content and more "maple" taste. The end of the season brings mostly Grade B, which was formerly known as Grade C, with even more minerals and the strongest maple flavor. All grades can be used in the diet but the darker grades are the most desirable. The grading system is based purely on the relative deepness of the amber coloring and has nothing to do with the quality of the syrup, which is generally about the same for all organically produced maple syrup.

The maple syrup has a large variety of minerals and vitamins. Naturally the mineral and vitamin content will vary according to the area where the trees grow and the mineral content of the soil. These are the minerals found in the average samples of pure maple syrup: Sodium, Potassium, Calcium, Magnesium, Manganese, Iron, Copper, Phosphorus, Sulfur, and Silicon. Vitamin A, B1, B2, B6, C and Pantothenic Acid (B5) are also present in the syrup. Information on the need and effect of these properties will be found in the Biochemistry in the back of the book, "Healing for the Age of Enlightenment".

Some uninformed operators of the sugaring of the maple syrup do use formaldehyde pellets in the process of tapping the trees but there are many more that don't. Search out and demand the kind not using formaldehyde. The Maple River Valley in Westby, Wisconsin does not use it. This is the kind I recommend.

Dozens of letters weekly, from around the world highly praise the many superior benefits of the lemonade diet. Thus, we must conclude that since it does so much for so many it is truly The Master Cleanser. The following is a quote from one of the letters: "I tried the lemonade diet with exceptionally beneficial results. I would like to order at least six at whatever your wholesale price would be -- I know I will need many more as I do push the books. I believe they are the best in their field."

An ideal formula involves freshly extracted juice from the sugar cane (readily available in India, but not generally in the United States at the present time):

10 oz. fresh sugar cane juice (medium hot or cold)
2 tbsp. fresh lime or lemon juice
1/10 tsp cayenne (red pepper) or to taste

Another possible but lesser replacement could be pure sorghum. It does not produce equal or close to the benefits of maple syrup.

What About the Use of Honey?

Honey must not be used at any time internally. It is manufactured from the nectar picked up from the flowers by the bees — good enough in itself, perhaps — then predigested, vomited and stored for their own future use with a preservative added. It is deficient in calcium and has many detrimental effects for the human being.

According to one authority, honey is "a magical and mystical word in Healthfoodland. It is one of the most overpromoted, overpriced product being sold to gullible health foodists. The great value attributed to honey is delusive . . . honey is only a little less empty and more dangerous than sugar."

Just as with alcohol, honey, being predigested, enters the blood directly, raising the sugar content very rapidly above normal. To correct this, the pancreas must produce insulin immediately or possible death can occur. More insulin than necessary is likely to be produced, and the blood sugar level then drops below normal. This can produce blackout spells and even death if it goes too low. When blood sugar is below normal, a person will feel depressed. The regular use of honey can create constant imbalances which in turn will adversely affect the normal function of the liver, pancreas and spleen. Hypoglycemia and hyperglycemia are the results of the use of unbalanced sugars. The balanced sugar in maple syrup and sugar cane juice causes no dangerous side effects. All natural fruits and vegetables have balanced sugars in them. Artificial, synthetic, and refined sugars have no place in a natural diet.

18

Blend a part of the lemon skin and pulp with the lemonade in a blender for further cleansing and laxative effect. (Note: commercially procured lemons may have had their skins dyed with yellow coloring and may have been subjected to poisonous insect sprays — be sure to peel off the outer skin if you cannot get uncolored, organically grown lemons.) The properties in the lemon skin also act as a hemostatic to prevent excess bleeding and to prevent clotting internally should there be any such prevailing condition. (Don't worry — normal conditions will continue during the menstrual periods.)

Adding the cayenne pepper is necessary as it breaks up mucus and increases warmth by building the blood for an additional lift. It also adds many of the B and C vitamins.

Mint tea may be used occasionally during this diet as a pleasant change and to assist further in the cleansing. Its chlorophyll helps as a purifier, neutralizing many mouth and body odors that are released during the cleansing period.

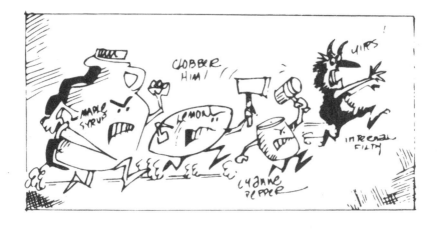

How Much Does One Drink?

Take from six to twelve glasses of the lemonade daily during the waking period. As you get hungry just have another glass of lemonade. NO OTHER FOOD SHOULD BE TAKEN DURING THE FULL PERIOD OF THE DIET. As this is a complete balance of minerals and vitamins, one does not suffer the pangs of hunger. Do not use vitamin pills. All solid food is turned into a liquid state before it can be carried by the blood to the cells of the body. The lemonade is already a food in liquid form.

For those who are overweight, less maple syrup may be taken. For those underweight, more maple syrup may be taken. For those who are underweight and worried about losing more weight, REMEMBER, the only things you can possibly lose are mucus, waste, and disease. Healthy tissue will not be eliminated. Many people who need to gain weight actually do so near the end of the diet period.

Never vary the amount of lemon juice per glass. About six glasses of lemonade a day is enough for those wishing to reduce. Extra water may be taken as desired.

Helping the Cleansing Along

As this is a cleansing diet, the more you can assist Nature to eliminate poisons, the better. **If your system feels upset, it is because you are not having sufficient elimination.** Avoid this possibility by following the directions completely. Above all, be sure you have two, three, or more movements a day. This may seem unnecessary not eating solid food, but it is Nature's way of eliminating the waste it has loosened from the various cells and organs in the body. They must leave the body some way. It would be just the same as sweeping the floor around and around and never removing the dirt from the house if the wastes were not passed out. The better the elimination, the more rapid will be the results.

A LAXATIVE HERB TEA is found to be the best helper for most persons. It is a good practice to take a good laxative herb tea right from the beginning — the last thing at night and first thing in the morning. There are several good laxative teas. They are best taken in a liquid form. Buy them in your health food store.

Another Cleansing Aid: Internal Salt Water Bathing

As it is necessary to bathe the outside of our bodies, so it is with the inside. Do not take enemas or colonics at any time during the cleansing diet or afterwards. They are unnecessary and can be extremely harmful.

There is a much superior method of cleansing the colonic tract without the harmful effects of customary colonics and enemas. This method will cleanse the entire digestive tract while the colonics and enemas will only reach the colon or a small part of it. Colonics can be expensive while our salt water method is not.

DIRECTIONS: Prepare a full quart of luke-warm water and add two level (rounded for the Canadian quart) teaspoons of uniodized sea salt. Do not use ordinary iodized salt as it will not work properly. Drink the entire quart of salt and water first thing in the morning. This must be taken on an empty stomach. The salt and water will not separate but will stay intact and quickly and thoroughly wash the entire tract in about one hour. Several eliminations will likely occur. The salt water has the same specific gravity as the blood, hence the kidneys cannot pick up the water and the blood cannot pick up the salt. This may be taken as often as needed for proper washing of the entire digestive system.

If the salt water does not work the first time, try adding a little more or a little less salt until the proper balance is found; or possibly take extra water with or without salt. This often increases the activity. Remember, it can do no harm at any time. The colon needs a good washing, but do it the natural way — the salt water way.

It is quite advisable to take the herb laxative tea at night to loosen, then the salt water each morning to wash it out. If for some reason the salt water cannot be taken in the morning, then the herb laxative tea must be taken night and morning.

Should I Take "Supplements"?

Some people want to take vitamin pills or food supplements while on the diet. This frequently fails to produce the desired result. There are many reasons. As the lymphatic glands become clogged, they are no longer able to assimilate and digest even the best of foods. As we cleanse our bodies and free our cells and glands of toxins that clog and paralyze our assimilation, we free our various organs and processes to do their proper jobs. Note Page 20. All the necessary vitamins and minerals are in the lemonade, and therefore we do not need an additional supply in most cases.

Vitamin pills and supplements do not grow on trees as such but rather come to us in fruits, berries, vegetables and plants. Man will never take a group of natural or synthetic foods; process and combine them in a variety of products, and come up with anything equal or better than the original. They have lost much of their basic life and energy by combining them according to a man made concept. Many dangerous side effects can occur because of improper and unequal balances present. Stay with the natural laws of balance. First one must decided if God is right or if man is right. If God is right then man and his ideas of processing — tearing apart and rearranging — are likely to be wrong.

Later, as we consume a more complete variety of foods, we find our sources of vitamins and minerals complete and in forms that are easily assimilated — it should not be necessary to return to these supplements even if one is accustomed to taking them. The sources of good food are steadily being enlarged as people become more educated concerning them. Search these sources and rely on them for your total nutritional needs.

The lemon is a loosening and cleansing agent with many important building factors. The ability of the elements in the lemon and the maple syrup working together creates these desired results.

Its 49% potassium strengthens and energizes the heart, stimulates and builds the kidneys and adrenal glands.

Its oxygen builds vitality.

Its carbon acts as a motor stimulant.

Its hydrogen activates the sensory nervous system.

Its calcium strengthens and builds the lungs.

Its phosphorus knits the bones, stimulates and builds the brain for clearer thinking.

Its sodium encourages tissue building.

Its magnesium acts as a blood alkalizer.

Its iron builds the red corpuscles to rapidly correct the most common forms of anemia.

Its chlorine cleanses the blood plasma.

Its silicon aids the thyroid for deeper breathing.

The natural iron, copper, calcium, carbon, and hydrogen found in the sweetening supplies more building and cleansing material. It truly is a perfect combination for cleansing, eliminating, healing, and building. Hence, supplements are not needed during the diet and may actually interfere with its cleansing action.

What About the Use of Vitamins?

Vitamins and minerals have always been a necessary part of natural living. Not satisfied with God's plan, man has attempted to improve the situation by separating them from fresh live foods, then processing and combining them to conform to his concept of what they should be. Not satisfied with the finished product, attempts were made to produce them synthetically. It was big business — and we became a world of "pill pushers," whether they were needed or not. More often they were not needed. No one really knew if the pills were needed, or how many — people just took them because they **might** have a deficiency!

Just how these vitamins and minerals should be balanced and formu-lated led to many differences of opinion. A large variety of experts, in processing and manufacturing of pills, disagree as to how the many billions of pills should be made. They all have different formulas and claim theirs are the best even though much is lost in the processing. However, even without any clear consensus as to their worth and use, they were manufactured and processed; therefore they must be sold with no thought as to possible side effects from overdosing or imbalances. Millions of dollars are made by the producers and the sellers with little regard for the true needs of the consumer.

In reality, the whole process could have been completely avoided. Our Creator has already done a better job of making sure we receive all the needed vitamins and minerals in a perfectly balanced form. Only the finest of natural foods in their original package are good enough for bringing complete energy and life to build and retain a healthy body. Any time man attempts to improve on God's formulas and plans, the result is bound to be a failure.

The simple rules to complete nutrition include all the vitamins and minerals needed by all mankind and all animals. Our Creator has given the right food for the right animal for complete nutrition. This is also true for man. When these foods are properly prepared and eaten, there is nothing more that man can do to prepare a better food.

As we eat the correct foods without excesses, the body will produce ALL the needed vitamins. Foods grown properly, in complete, mineral-rich soil, will have all the minerals in them. Thus, we have no need for vitamin enriched foods, created synthetically by man, nor for extra minerals.

All refined and devitalized foods must be completely eliminated from our diet. If refined and devitalized foods are eaten, then and only then does man have any need for additional supplements. Just how much and what combination, even with long and complicated tests, will probably never be determined, so this form of unnatural nutrition will always be lacking. Such a plan is a very poor substitute for the right way.

Will It Make Me Feel Bad or Weak?

In the cleansing process, some people experience a tremendous stirring up and may even feel worse for several days. It is not the lemonade that causes the trouble, but what the lemonade stirs up in the system that causes our dizziness and other disturbances. Vomiting may occur under certain conditions; increased pain may be felt in the various joints of the body; dizziness may develop on certain days. If weakness develops at any time, it is the result of poisons circulating through the blood stream rather than a lack of food or vitamins. This diet gives a person all the vitamins, food, and energy necessary for the full ten days or longer in a liquid form. Rest and take it a little easier if you have to — although most people can go on about their regular business without difficulty. Keep right on with the diet; don't give up or "cheat" by eating a little food or you may destroy the benefits.

Even though the lemon is an acid fruit, it becomes alkaline as it is digested and assimilated. It is, in fact, our best aid toward proper alkaline balance. There is no danger of "too much acid."

Alcoholics, smokers, and other drug addicts will receive untold benefits from this diet. The chemical changes and the cleansing have a way of removing the craving and the many probable deficiencies. Thus the desire for the unnatural types of stimulants and depressants disappears. The usual cravings experienced and suffered in breaking away from drugs, alcohol, and tobacco no longer present themselves during and after this diet.

It is truly a wonderful feeling to be free from slavery to these many habit-forming and devitalizing elements of modern living. Coffee, tea, and various cola drinks, as habit-forming beverages, also lose their appeal through the marvels of the lemonade diet.

How to Break the Lemonade Diet

Coming off the lemonade diet properly is highly important — please follow the directions very carefully. After living in a semi-tropical and tropical climate for many years, I find that people have increasingly turned to a raw fruit, nut, and vegetable diet. Following is the schedule for people who normally follow such a natural vegetarian diet:

FIRST and SECOND DAY AFTER DIET:
Several 8 oz. glasses of fresh orange juice as desired during the day. The orange juice prepares the digestive system to properly digest and assimilate regular food. Drink it slowly. If there has been any digestive difficulty prior to or during the change over, extra water may be taken with the orange juice.

THIRD DAY:
Orange juice in the morning. Raw fruit for lunch. Fruit or raw vegetable salad at night. You are now ready to eat normally.

For those who have characteristically lived the unnatural way of meat, milk, refined and devitalized food, it may be best to change over as follows, gradually adopting the raw fruit, nut, and vegetable diet:

FIRST DAY:
Several 8 oz. glasses of fresh orange juice as desired during the day.
Drink it slowly.

SECOND DAY:
Drink several 8 oz. glasses of orange juice during the day — with
extra water, if needed. Some time during the afternoon prepare a
vegetable soup (no canned soup) as follows:

Recipe for Vegetable Soup

Use several kinds of vegetables, perhaps one or two kinds
of legumes, potatoes, celery, carrots, green vegetable tops,
onion, etc. Dehydrated vegetables or vegetable soup powders
may be added for extra flavor. Okra or okra powder, chili,
curry, cayenne (red) pepper, tomatoes, green peppers, and
zucchini squash may be included to good advantage. Brown
rice may be used, but no meat or meat stock. Other spices may
be added (delicately) for flavor. Use salt delicately as a limited
amount of salt is necessary. Learn to enjoy the natural flavor of
the vegetables. The less cooking the better. Read the special
article on salt in the September 1977 issue of National Geog-
raphic magazine.

Have this soup for the evening meal using the broth mostly, although
some of the vegetables may be eaten. Rye wafers may be eaten
sparingly with the soup, but no bread or crackers.

THIRD DAY:
Drink orange juice in the morning. At noon have some more soup;
enough may be made the night before and put in the refrigerator. For
the evening meal eat whatever is desired in the form of vegetables,
salads, or fruit. No meat, fish, or eggs; no bread, pastries, tea, coffee,
or milk. Milk is highly mucus-forming and tends to develop toxins
throughout the body.
(Milk, being a predigested food, has been known to cause various
complications in the stomach and colon, such as cramps and
convulsions. The calcium in milk is difficult to assimilate and may
cause toxins in the form of rheumatic fever, arthritis, neuritis, and
bursitis. The resulting lack of proper digestion and assimilation of

the calcium allows it to go into the blood stream in a free form and it is deposited in the tissues, cells, and joints where it can cause intense pain and suffering.)

FOURTH DAY:
Normal eating may be resumed, but best health will be retained if the morning meal consists of our type of lemonade or fruit juice; and, of course, if a strictly fruit, vegetable, seed and berry diet is followed. If, after eating is resumed, distress or gas occurs, it is suggested that the lemonade diet be continued for several more days until the system is ready for food.

Recap of the steps to be taken in the diet. Be careful to read the entire instructions so that the diet will be of the best benefit to you.

First prepare yourself mentally to follow in detail the entire directions and continue as long as is needed to make the necessary changes. One of the best signals of the completed diet is when the formerly coated and fuzzy tongue is clear pink and clean looking. During the diet it becomes very badly coated.

The Night Before starting the diet take the laxative tea.

In the morning take the salt water (or) laxative tea (see page 18 for details). This should be done each night and morning during the diet — rare exception — if diarrhea develops. When diarrhea is ended then continue above directions.

Now the lemonade formula

Breaking the diet. Be absolutely sure you follow the directions very carefully to prepare your body for normal eating (our way). Do not over eat or eat too soon. Serious problems (nausea) can occur if detailed directions are not followed.

How Do I Get My Protein?

Often the question is asked about the need for amino acids, and animal protein foods. The need is highly exaggerated as only 16% of our body is protein. The answer to the question is very simple. We first need to understand that pure protein is primarily nitrogen, with oxygen, hydrogen and some carbon. We all know we get a large share of our oxygen and hydrogen needs from the air along with some carbon. There is four times the amount of nitrogen in the same air as there is oxygen, hydrogen and carbon combined. Since we are able to utilize and assimilate a large amount of our needs of these elements into our bodies we are able to assimilate and build the nitrogen also into our bodies as protein. This is done by natural bacteria action which is capable of converting it to our use.

From the combination of the best of foods and clean air we are able to create our own amino acids, just as well as the animals do. We never try to feed amino acids to the animals. Thus we are able to eliminate the need for toxic dead animal flesh and have no further need to worry about our constant source of protein. Eat only the best variety of fruits, berries, nuts, vegetables, seeds and sprouted seeds for a further complete source of protein.

People who smoke cannot pick up the nitrogen from the air so easily, but will still get enough from proper food without the use of animal flesh. For your well being, however, elimination of smoking is a must.

Many people believe that eating meat gives them strength. If this is so, then why are the strongest animals in the world vegetarians? Did you ever stop to think that the animals you do eat are vegetarian? Where did they get their strength? All the meat-eating animals find it necessary to sleep 16 to 18 hours daily because of excess toxins. The meat eating animals live a very short life. God has supplied such a bountiful supply of fresh, wholesome food that there is never a need to kill an animal for its more toxic flesh in our modern civilization.

Feeding Your Baby

All babies should be nursed by the mother if at all possible. There is no real substitute. Cows and goats milk is for their babies and is not suitable for the human baby. It creates mucus and other problems just the same as in adults, including colds and infectious diseases.

Correct food, reflex stimulation, and color therapy will assure the mother all the milk she needs for her baby. Where mother's milk is not available the best replacement is coconut milk — see recipe on page 33. With this, give the baby about 8 ounces of lemonade in between regular feedings. To the regular formula for lemonade add about double the amount of water until the infant is about six months old and then gradually change to regular strength. A nursing baby should begin to be weaned in nine months and be eating regular foods after that.

Commercially prepared baby foods and baby formulas are unfit for the balanced need of a healthy baby. Recent articles and TV reports indicate these foods are very undesirable **always.** Prepare fresh food from fruit, vegetables, berries, and seeds. The baby has no need for any of the animal or fish products. Use pure maple syrup instead of sugar or honey when sweetening is needed. Your baby deserves only the very best of live fresh foods. Caring for a healthy baby is a great pleasure with fewer problems when this pattern is followed. At the same time it develops good lifelong habits of sound nutrition.

Is Water Fasting a Good Thing?

The subject of water fasting often presents itself. I am very much opposed to several days or weeks of water fasting. It is too dangerous and is unnecessary to achieve the desired results of internal cleansing.

Many people are already deficient as well as toxic. The longer they do without food, the greater becomes the deficiency. The lemonade diet can more than match all the possible good obtained from fasting and at the same time will rebuild any possible deficiency.

Ordinarily with fasting it is necessary to take it easy by resting or staying in bed. On the contrary, with the lemonade diet there is no need to become a useless member of society — you may live an active, normal life. Many workers at hard labor have found they are able to do more and harder work while on the lemonade diet than on their normal diet.

After one has attained a clean, healthy body, and then desires to fast for purely spiritual reasons, thirty or even forty days can cause no harm. First we must build our physical bodies to their highest condition.

Your friends and acquaintances may find this lemonade diet to be the answer to their aches, pains, or other troubles. Even if there appears to be nothing wrong, sometimes those who are "never sick" will feel even better. Let your friends receive this benefit too.

A Gift of Life to Sheila

Around the year of 1958 we gave a class in Hemet, California. A Mr. & Mrs. C. were in this class. During the next few years they accomplished many wonderful things in healing. One of their most outstanding cases would stand out as truly a miracle in any field or system of healing.

Some time in 1963 Mr. C. took on the responsibility of raising and caring for his great niece at the age of 3½ weeks. She was diagnosed by the medical doctor as hopeless and beyond any form of help to his knowledge. He expected her to die within a few days. There was nothing medicine had to offer as a life saver. He told the parents "Take her home

29

and enjoy her for a few days as she has not long to live."

The couple accepting the responsibility, proceeded to feed and care for her with natural methods. The feeding consisted of fresh lemonade, orange juice and carrot juice for about three years. Gradually she was fed other natural raw foods — no animal milk or processed foods. Treatments consisted of the color therapy and Vita-Flex as a part of the healing and building process.

I had the special privilege of seeing this girl at the age of 14 years. The beauty and the poise of the girl was most outstanding. She is now an accomplished organist, pianist, opera singer and artist in painting.

She was raised without any form of animal products and has never had any form of medication, operation or shots. Also during these 14 years she has had none of the diseases that other children have when raised by the orthodox methods.

Sheila came to me at our first meeting and stated rather emotionally, "Mr. Burroughs, you have no idea how much we appreciate you — because without you and your system I could not have lived."

At that moment I thought to myself how wonderful that through my strong and constant desire I had created a system that had saved her life and could save the life of many other hopeless cases like hers if only the entire world knew about it.

Suddenly all of the countless years of frustrations I had encountered in producing this work seemed to disappear and this made everything all worth while. The thrill of knowing and using this knowledge to bring life more abundant to a suffering world knows no bounds.

This case, like many other cases prove that, when we work knowingly with all the natural laws, diseases, as we know them, no longer exist. This work must go on and be available to everyone no matter who or where they are.

A New Treatment for an Old Ailment: DROPSY (EDEMA)

Dropsy is one of the most difficult and least understood of the many expressions of toxemia. It consists of a accumulation of fluid in the body tissues. Varied attempts to correct this condition have met with little or no success. The main treatments can give only temporary relief and the final result, as these treatments fail to produce any change, is death from internal drowning.

To achieve fast relief and lasting correction, one must completely understand the causes. Then our unusual and simple approach to an ancient disease will achieve quick and lasting results.

As with so many other diseases, dropsy represents a vast accumulation of toxic wastes. These toxins accumulate because our eliminative organs are unable to take care of them as fast as they enter or are formed in the body. As accumulations steadily increase, they first appear to us in liquid form. If they are not eliminated from our body, they are automatically and gradually dehydrated or crystallized. They are then deposited in any and all of the available spaces throughout our cells, glands, and organs. This continues until a saturation point is reached and then Nature reverses the action and slowly dissolves the crystallized and dehydrated material. This change is the body's final effort to save the life from being snuffed out from complete stoppage of all glands and organs. Only in a liquid or semi-liquid form can we eliminate our toxins. Usually, by this time our eliminative organs are overworked and clogged, our heart, liver, and kidneys suffering the most, so they cannot carry off the liquid toxins. The body then steadily increases in size until it can no longer sustain life.

The correction for this otherwise fatal condition is simple, fast, and effective. Just follow directions and the results will be most satisfactory.

Now, the treatment. Start the patient off on the lemonade diet. This begins the internal cleansing process.

Next, secure one hundred (100) pounds of coarse rock salt (which may be purchased at a feed store). Cover the bottom of the bath tub with about two inches of salt. Unclothe the patient and wrap the person in a wet sheet. Then lay the patient on the salt and add salt to about two inches above their body so that the entire body is surrounded with the salt. The room should be 80° or slightly higher so the patient does not get chilled. (The tub may be warmed first with hot water before adding the salt. Let ALL the water out first before adding the salt.)

Leave the patient in the salt for approximately one hour. Be sure you have given them several glasses of hot lemonade with cayenne pepper in advance.

Remove the patient from the salt and wrap them in a woolen blanket to keep them warm. Extra heat may be used if necessary. Repeat this treatment every other day or daily, if not too weak from the rapid changes.

This may be repeated until all the swelling has gone down or the toxins are removed. The first application may not produce notable results. but from then on a rapid change should be observed.

31

Be sure to keep the dropsy victim on the lemonade diet until a big change has taken place, even if it continues for ten, twenty, or thirty days. Color and Vita-Flex may be used also and will provide tremendously increased action and elimination.

IMPORTANT NOTE: The salt may be used over and over on the same patient, but not on any other. Each person must have their own salt.

Bathing one or two times a day, especially during this diet, is especially necessary. We eliminate wastes through the breathing, the skin, the kidneys, the colon and from the sinus through the nose. The most wastes are eliminated by breathing; next in order are the skin, the colon, the kidneys, and depending on the individual, from the sinus. Often we eliminate large quantities of wastes in the form of mucus as we develop colds or flu. One can see how important becomes our elimination by the skin. Even when in good condition, it is important to bathe once or twice daily to remove these wastes from the surface of the skin, thus allowing it to breathe properly. These baths will help to eliminate obnoxious odors while we cleanse our body. Frequent steam baths will also help.

The Simple Art of Nutrition

There are simple, well-defined laws or rules to follow to obtain the utmost from the preparation and use of foods.These laws are natural, easily understood, and readily demonstrated.

Only when we follow these laws and live within their simplicity does our blood become pure and our minds serene. As we live within these simple laws we can dismiss all thoughts of disease, and it will never be necessary to seek help or relief from any outside source.

This excellent health has been achieved in thousands of cases involving every variety of disease condition. All diseases and adverse conditions respond and disappear as we discover the healthy way.

Cleansing, building, and retaining is the master plan of this simple form of nutrition. Before building and retaining can be realized, cleansing of the various toxins, poisons, and congestions must be complete.

I offer you the finest in the cleansing and healing field in the form of the lemonade diet.

In an article in the **National Enquirer,** July 22, 1975, there was the following prediction by Jeanne Dixon: "One of the greatest medical breakthroughs of the decade will come from the common citrus fruit. Scientists will create fantastic new wonder drugs from these fruits for a wide array of illnesses that have plagued mankind for centuries. It will be learned that a chemical in the fruit can strengthen our natural resistance to many diseases."

In reality, the chemical or chemicals present in the citrus do not actually make the body resistant to disease; rather, they eliminate the causes of disease by their cleansing action. These fantastic new wonder chemicals have already been discovered many years ago by me, and they are already being used in the form of the lemonade diet with tremendous success around the world.

There is no need to further create these chemicals as God has already done a better job of it than any group of men can ever hope to do, regardless of their education or abilities. These chemicals are already in the citrus fruit to function at the highest level of efficiency because other necessary chemicals are present with them. As various chemicals are separated or isolated, unbalances, resulting in harmful side effects can occur, defeating the original plan to cleanse and build. Only when we use the best of foods in their **original form,** are we going to get the most out of them.

For many years I have been telling my students that we always need the whole product instead of the various separated units such as carrot juice, vegetable juices, etc. We throw away the pulp — fibre — and take only the juice. There are many needed properties in the fibre also to assist in properly handling the juices. Is it not feasable that the lack of them can cause deficiences or unbalances? We know from excellent results that carrot juice, celery juice and other vegetable juices are excellent but how much better can they be if left intact and taken as is. Can we possibly get as much good and complete nutrition from drinking a dozen carrots without the fibre as we can from properly chewing the whole carrot and eating fewer carrots.

Recent findings tell us that fibre "is that important". Formerly we were told not to use fibre as it might cause a variety of colon troubles. In determining this importance and putting it to use should we go over board with the idea by using such things as wood fiber in bread, (good for termites but not much good for us) or say cereal, or perhaps some other foreign matter in these products or should we use it as it is originally without separating it in the first place. Reminds me of the white bread controversy — tests showed that white bread could not sustain life even though milk and eggs had been added so a variety of vitamins were added — enriched — fortified flour they called it. Then new standards were found or believed to be necessary so more enrichments were added — then extra iron — extra spoilage retardants or preservatives appeared necessary — next extra fiber was found that important. Now after all these things were added just how good was the bread — taking things out and adding other things to replace them. Could they be as good as the original ingredients? White bread has always seemed like a sickly looking mess to me. Surely there is a reason for the bulk and other things being there originally. Perhaps they figured God made a mistake so man must correct it.

The whole matter could have been prevented by leaving things as they were originally. Now if we can accept the whole procedure as a much needed lesson we can then leave the rest of our food as it is and stop taking extra wheat germ, lecithin, vitamins, minerals, fibre (bran or wood) and many other extras to supplement and enrich a large variety of separated and devitalized products.

Another thought by so many people "If a small amount is good: then logic tells them that a lot can do so much more". By taking a lot more isn't it possible that again we might be going overboard and consuming more than the body can handle at one time so we must then work overtime to handle and eliminate the excess or hopelessly clog up the works and defeat our original reason for following the procedures. Then there is the pulp — bulk — which is left out. Something is left out so what deficiences have we created and what about the following side effects.

It seems to me we should start all over again from the beginning: start eating things as they are in limited amounts to allow the body to digest and assimilate just the amount it can handle with no excesses.

The use of a high protein for weight reducing became a fad and then a predigested protein is creating many serious deficiencies and developed a monster to the point that it was reported that many have died from lack of potassium, and other needed life qualities.

This simple idea can and will save us a lot of time, money and useless research to test for possible deficiences. Certainly the monetary saving advantages can become a major importance.

The ideal purpose of any complete diet is to have all the vitamins, minerals, and nutrients in a readily available form in order to enable the body to function normally and to be free from diseases and other malfunctions.

Since many people of the world are already handicapped by a multiplicity of diseases, they must first cleanse the body before the right diet can be properly used. Thus, the sick and suffering must first turn to the best of all cleansing diets, THE MASTER CLEANSER or LEMONADE DIET.

MENU SUGGESTIONS

Our system goes through a cleansing process from twelve midnight until twelve noon, and a building program from twelve noon to twelve midnight. Therefore, what is eaten during these respective periods must be harmonious with the natural processes. The following suggestions take this natural process into account.

BREAKFAST: Nothing more is required by the body than fresh lemonade, fresh orange or grapefruit juice. Occasionally, if one has no desire for even this, try some hot peppermint tea. It gives a clean feeling and is a wonderful tonic.

NOON LUNCH: Lunch may be omitted with no ill effects; many will find a small amount of fruit entirely sufficient. If one desires more, a small vegetable or fruit salad may be eaten. Soup (homemade, vegetarian, of course) or tomato juice, hot or cold, may be taken with vegetable salad. Coconut milk or almond milk may be taken with the fruit salad.

Note: Recipes for coconut and almond milk, and for a number of dressings, are to be found on the following pages.

DINNER (Evening): Simple preparation of dinner involves starting with a vegetable soup, then having two or three vegetables steamed slightly. On other occasions try special dishes such as vegetable stew, various types of brown rice dishes (curried rice, Spanish rice, chop suey and rice), chili beans (made with lima beans or red beans), or any recipe using lentils or garbanzos — but no meat, of course. Vegetarian cutlets, and all similar commercially-produced meat substitute preparations, should be used very, very sparingly, or not at all.

All kinds of berries are an excellent addition for both lunch and dinner.

Change your menu daily. Be sure there is plenty of variety from day to day. Do not over eat — stick to small portions. An occasional mono diet meal is always beneficial such as brown rice with coconut milk and a little maple syrup only, steamed artichokes only, fresh green corn only, watermellon, strawberries, honeydew. Many other single items can readily come to mind.

The accepted idea of five necessary categories of foods daily is quite faulty. It is very time consuming, costly and does not accomplish the desired results that simplification can. Different types of foods have different requirement in time and abilities to properly digest them. Too many combinations often cause a variety of digestive disturbances.

COCONUT MILK

Coconut milk may be used in all recipes calling for milk. Other nut milks are also good. They are superior and preferred to the use of any of the animal milks. Use fresh nuts in preference to canned or grated nuts. To prepare coconut milk, start with liquefier (blender) ½ full of warm water. Add 2 tbsp. of maple syrup and a dash of salt. (These two ingredients may be left out if not desired.)

As liquefier is running (medium to high speed) add chunks of coconut until container is nearly full. (Dried coconut may be used.)

Strain the pulp from the liquid and use the pulp over again by adding fresh warm water to it in the blender. Strain again, and this time throw the used pulp away.

The coconut milk produced in this fashion makes a tasty, nutritious beverage for children or adults in place of animal milk. A number of delicious drinks can be made by using coconut milk and your favorite fresh fruit liquefied together.

COCONUT-SESAME MIX
(May be used for many cream sauces.)

6 tbsp. grated coconut
6 tbsp. fresh sesame seeds
Sesame or safflower oil

Liquify the two dry ingredients until they no longer fall to center. Stop the blender and push them to the center with a knife several times as they stick to the sides.

As liquefier is running add sesame or safflower oil until the oil covers the pulp (approx. 6 tbsp.). Liquefy for 2 minutes and then add warm water until mixture reaches the desired thickness (approx. 12 oz. of water). One tbsp. of maple syrup and a dash of salt may be added if desired.

FOR SAUCES: Start with coconut milk, or coconut-sesame milk; add potato flour for thickening and season with desired spices. May also be used for creamed soups (mushroom, celery, etc.) and scalloped dishes (potato, cauliflower, etc.) Try variations as your imagination dictates.

ALMOND MILK

Start with 1 lb. of shelled almonds (dry) in the blender. Blend until they no longer fall to the center. Push them to the center with a knife several times as they stick to the side as the blender is running. Add sesame or safflower oil until pulp is covered (approximately 7 tbsp.) Blend for 2 minutes more and then add warm water until mixture is desired thickness. Two to three glasses of water should be sufficient. One or two tbsp. of maple syrup and a dash of salt may be added if desired.

This makes a nice drink or may be used for any milk recipe.

MAYONNAISE

Start with the coconut-sesame milk, but keep it medium thick by using less than the customary water. Add the following:

5 tbsp. apple cider vinegar
1 tbsp. maple syrup
2 cloves garlic
1 tsp. paprika
1 tsp. chili powder
1 tsp. powdered mustard
1 tsp. turmeric
½ tsp. sweet basil
Salt to taste

VEGETABLE SALAD DRESSING No. 1

Using preceding mayonnaise dressing to start add extra spices, delicately, such as dill seed, curry powder, cayenne pepper, fennel seed, or oregano. A couple of dill pickles and sweet relish may be added to provide the Thousand Island taste.

VEGETABLE SALAD DRESSING No. 2

¾ cup olive, sesame, or safflower oil
½ cup vinegar (apple cider or wine)
2 tbsp. lemon or lime juice
3 tbsp. maple syrup
½ tsp. paprika
2 tsp. mustard
1 tsp. sweet basil
1 tsp. dill seed
½ tsp. cardamom
2 cloves garlic
2 tbsp. potato flour (optional)

Blend the oil and vinegar together first with the maple syrup, then add the other ingredients. Add the potato flour as needed if you desire the dressing to be thicker and creamier.

Other herbs and spices may be used very delicately instead of the suggested ones to create a variety of dressings.

FRENCH DRESSING

To the mayonnaise dressing add one good sized tomato or 1 cup tomato juice.

FRUIT SALAD DRESSING

Start with the basic coconut-sesame milk, then add:

½ cup maple syrup
2 ripe bananas
1 cup pineapple pieces (fresh if possible)

Nutmeg and cinnamon may be added for extra flavor.

COLE SLAW DRESSING No. 1

Start with the basic mayonnaise dressing and add:

1 tsp. dill seed
4 tbsp. vinegar
½ tsp. fennel seed

COLE SLAW DRESSING No. 2

¼ cup oil (cold pressed)
¼ tsp. powdered cloves
¼ tsp. ginger
¼ cup maple syrup
¼ cup apple cider vinegar
Salt
Juice of whole lemon
2 slices pineapple (¾" x 4")
2-3 tbsp. potato flour

Liquefy above ingredients, except potato flour, for 5 minutes. Slowly add potato flour as liquefier is running until desired thickness is achieved.

WHITE SAUCE

2 tbsp. margarine or vegetable oil
2 tbsp. potato or brown rice flour
Hot Water

Melt the margarine in a sauce pan. Stir in the potato or rice flour. Continue stirring as you add hot water until you have the desired thickness (approx. 1 cup). Salt as desired.

VARIATIONS OF WHITE SAUCE

1. To the white sauce add 1 tsp. each cardamom and coriander. The cardamon and coriander can be increased — even doubled to improve the taste.
2. Leave out the water and add one 8 oz. can of tomato sauce and ½ tsp. sweet basil.

CHAPTER III:

Special Needs and Problems

Special Hints

The following hints encompass some of the best of the simple and natural aids which are of great benefit in the correction of various minor inconveniences that may develop at any time in our lives.

Oil of Clove

Oil of clove is invaluable for many things. It is especially good for skin cancers, warts, and corns. With the finger, apply a small amount on warts or corns. Wait a short time. With an emery stick, scrape the top off and apply oil again. Repeat this several times daily until wart or corn disappears. Do the same thing for skin cancer. These forms of blemishes are not caused by a virus, but are a form of fungus growth feeding on acid elimination in the skin. (Our type of diet, incidentally, prevent these conditions from forming in the beginning.)

Clove oil stops the pain in the following conditions:

Use a small amount on the gums for toothache, and swollen or sore parts of the mouth. Use for canker sores.

Use for all insect stings and bites (wasp and mosquito, for example), scratches, small burns, and sores that are slow in healing. It is an excellent disinfectant. It takes the sting out of nettles and poison oak.

Use your finger to put a small amount on the back of the tongue for sore throat or a tickling cough.

For those who wish to quite smoking — every time you have the desire for a smoke place — with your finger — a small amount on back of the tongue and you immediately lose your desire to smoke. This is the easy way if you really want to quit.

Bay Rum

Bay Rum makes a nice after shave lotion. The benefits received from Bay Rum are many. For infections, irritations, and itching inside the ear dip a Q-tip in the solution and place inside the ear for immediate relief. Use as often as needed with no side effects.

For dandruff and itchy scalp — use straight and rub into the scalp.

For all irritations on the skin surfaces it is very healing. It brings fast relief to irritated parts in the groin.

Use as an astrigent for the face and neck — very refreshing. Also helps to relieve sunburn and chapped skin.

Camphor and Camphor Cubes

When taking a bath in a tub, place 2 camphor cubes in the water. It is an excellent skin softener and relieves itching.

Camphor liniment is excellent for tired and sore muscles. It is a super skin conditioner. It relieves itching and pain of insect bites.

Camphor makes an excellent inhalent. It clears the head.

Castor Oil

Castor oil is fine for corns, warts, and other skin blemishes.

Coconut Oil

Coconut is one of the finest oils for the skin. It softens, removes wrinkles, and adds body to the skin. It helps to prevent sunburn and windburn. It is a fine dressing for the hair.

Honey

While honey does more harm than good internally (see page 15), it is especially good for many conditions externally. It heals many kinds of sores. It is very good for infections and in poultices.

Osage Rub

Osage Rub is an excellent commercial product for tired and sore muscles and skin. It is very cooling and refreshing. It makes an ideal after shave lotion. On a warm day, rub a small amount on the face and neck as a cooling agent.

Peppermint Oil

Peppermint oil is excellent for headaches. It clears the sinus. It cools and refreshes to enable free breathing. Place a small amount on one hand (tip the bottle upside down with the palm tight against the opening). Rub the two palms together and then inhale through the nose and mouth for a short time. Later, place the palms on forehead and back of the head. It is very cooling — especially helpful in case of fevers. A small amount of peppermint on the finger and rubbed inside the mouth makes the mouth feel refreshed and cool.

Wintergreen

The true oil of Wintergreen is superior to the synthetic, so use it if possible. The synthetic will work, but not as well.

It relieves pain in warts and corns. It is an excellent product for sore and painful muscles and joints. It is very warming — increasing circulation.

Witch Hazel

Witch Hazel is an excellent astringent and skin conditioner. It is a natural for an after shave application. It gives fast relief for sore and irritated skin all over the body.

Vinegar

Pure Apple Cider Vinegar is a simple and safe, natural antibiotic. It may be used on the outside or inside of the body. If used on the outside, full strength is completely safe. If used on the inside, it must be diluted.

Athletes Foot: Four to five days of frequent use on feet will clear the condition. Use it periodically from then on to prevent a return. Works faster than other medication.

Chapped Sore Hands: Any fungus condition on hands or other parts of the body, is quickly corrected with straight vinegar.

Dandruff: Straight vinegar on the head clears dandruff very quickly.

Ring Worm: (on any part of the body): Vinegar often does the job of stopping it. Often stronger methods are necessary. For these occasions, pure peppermint oil works well. If this is not available, a commercial product called "Heet" works very well. The more frequently these products are applied, the faster the condition disappears.

Sore Throat: Vinegar and water — half and half — is an excellent gargle for sore throat and to cut mucus. It is also excellent for canker sores and infections or swellings in the mouth.

Indigestion or Gas: 2 teaspoons of vinegar in a glass of water; may be consumed with the meal or any time afterwards as needed. Use the same amount to stop dysentary or diarrhea — take it every hour until the condition has cleared. However, diarrhea can be very helpful for cleaning and eliminating of surplus toxins from the body. Do not be in too big a rush to stop the body's natural process in the cleansing.

Household uses: A vinegar application will loosen a rusted or corroded bolt.

For clearing stopped up sink pour ½ cup of baking soda down the drain. Add ½ glass of vinegar and cover for a minute.

Two tablespoons of vinegar and 2 tablespoons of maple syrup to a quart of water will aid in keeping cut flowers longer.

½ cup of ammonia and 3 tablespoons of vinegar added to each quart of warm water is excellent for washing windows without leaving film or streaks.

Special Formula for Eye Drops

This formula has been used with most excellent results for many years with absolutely no dangerous side effects when coupled with a change of diet, the reflex work and color therapy. Many cases of glaucoma, cataracts, spots, film, and growths of various kinds have completely disappeared. The drops may be applied one at a time to both eyes several times daily. Continue use until the condition is cleared up. Many people have completely overcome the necessity for glasses. In all cases eyes have improved greatly. There are a number of books written on eye exercises; their systems help greatly to bring the sight back to normal. Most people would do well to learn and perform exercises to insure the retention of normal vision.

Formula: 5 parts (measures) distilled water
2 parts best grade of honey
1 part pure apple cider vinegar
(Sterling or other good brand)

Mix together and store in a bottle. It need not be refrigerated as contents will not spoil. If eyes are in good condition, keep them that way by regular use as no harm can ever come by using it. It has a strong smarting effect for a moment, then the eyes clear and feel very good after each use. These drops have proven to be superior to most commercial drops.

Massage and Skin Conditioner.

All of the different oils and solutions may be added together to make one of the finest massage solutions available. Each ingredient compliments and aids the other to do a remarkable job for most above conditions.

Into a gallon container add:

1 pt. Bay rum
1 pt. Witch Hazel
3 pt. Rubbing alcohol
2 pt. water
2 tbsp. Camphor Liniment
1 tbsp. Oil of Clove
3 oz. Osage Rub
1 oz. Castor oil
2 oz. Heet (a commercial product)
1 oz. Apple Cider Vinegar
4 oz. Good Hand and Body Cream
2 oz. Honey (optional)
¼ oz. Eucalyptus
¼ oz. Peppermint Oil
¼ oz. Wintergreen Oil

Mix all together and use straight at any time for a most beneficial and refreshing tonic for the face and skin. These ingredients may be found in a drug store or barber supply.

The Abuse of Drugs

To descend to the bottom of the pit is the hard way to find that this is not the path to the heavenly bliss that one may have heard so much about. Many young people have sincerely sought "instant samadhi" through drugs, only to discover too late it was an abortive route. The many "drug abuse clinics" and "rehabilitation centers", engaged in piecing together the shattered and fragmented lives of our youth, are a symbol of our age.

The need for drugs of any kind has been greatly exaggerated. The over-development, manufacture, and sale of these drugs has systematically created a world of unnecessary addiction. The freedom with which these drugs are used staggers the imagination. For the most part, use of drugs has been minimal throughout history. It took modern chemistry, medicine, and greed, for profits and power to create a monster of addiction and suffering. The drugs that were used to relieve suffering, created misery and suffering by addiction.

Not wanting to be left out, the younger generation has understandably taken everything and anything they could get their little fingers into and made a big thing of it. Having no more common sense or control than adults, much damage to their bodies and minds has resulted. Crime, loss of property and life, has steadily increased with the increase in the use of these drugs.

Getting even, or striking back at our parents and the adult world in general, for their imperfections and lack of understanding is the hard way to prove a point. It only adds more problems to both parties involved. Must one become involved in the weaknesses and depravity of adult civilization in the entirely justifiable search for freedom?

The price we pay for this abuse has reached and gone beyond our ability to pay for and live with it. The trend must be reversed. The development, growth, and manufacture of these useless addictives must be eliminated from our society, if we ever hope to produce a better world to live in. Only when we create it can we ever hope to live in a better world.

Any possible good that drugs have to offer can easily be duplicated and improved upon by simple and natural methods. If these drugs were not manufactured and distributed by unscrupulous people in the adult world, there would be no possible way our children could procure them.

It is time for the younger generation to completely review the whole situation. It is the duty of the young and the vital to bring about the needed changes in our society. Why wait for the next generation? This creative renewal cannot be accomplished by wallowing in the filth the older generations have created. Don't let someone's greed for money and power be your downfall.

Drugs do not bring one closer to the Divine or free one from those imaginary shackles. As the effect of the drugs wear off, the old problems are still unsolved and new ones have been added. Drugs separate the psychic body from the physical. It is most difficult for the soul to remain healthy while the body is sick with drugs. While the psychic body is out of the physical, many adverse conditions can occur. Protective controls are gone, leaving the body wide open to destructive forces or lower spirit entities.

Leaving the body under such adverse conditions brings our psychic into an imaginary world of illusion or to the bottom of the pit of utter confusion. Any point there, or in between, can destroy the physical and leave us stranded in the world of confusion which only delays our journey to the higher realms of being. Heaven, God, or the finer things in life are not found in the doping and supressing of the physical body.

The drug way is surely the hard way to find reality. Keeping the mind and body free from the degrading effect of drugs gives it a strong incentive to advance more rapidly to the most desired form of living.

The natural way is the decision factor to be rid of all diseases. The Universal One would have it no any other way.

Within the light of Universal knowing all realities become evident.

Without the light of the Universal One, there is not much to look foreward to.

Medicine has struggled unsuccessfully for over two years for all the right answers as the sick and dying found little cause for respect for those they trusted so hopefully.

The Medical way has no resemblance to the natural way of the Universal One for freedom from all diseases.

THE HUMAN COMPUTER

A woman becomes pregnant and immediately the divine intelligence within takes over and a baby is formed. The woman has no control as to where the different parts are placed. It is all directed automatically by the divine computer within the mother and the newly developing mortal.

To many people, God seems so far away.
If so — who did the moving?

Within the human computer there is stored complete data that is constantly on the alert to diagnose and prescribe what is needed and where it should go to correct the damage or supply the deficiency in any part or parts. The computer requires only the best cooperation of each individual to supply the raw materials designed by nature to fill the need.

The ability of the computer is strictly and completely automatic giving complete directions for every part to act in accordance with nature to serve unfaulteringly to every need.

It is only when people ignore the simple natural needs of the body and become involved with drugs of any nature — legal or illegal — and a variety of denatured foods with excesses of any kind that people will become sick and crippled.

Even the computer will attempt to adjust and correct to the best of it's ability with what is given it to work with.

All form of illness reflect on the inability of it's host to supply it's needs rather than failure of the computer to perform to its desired perfection.

All the above completely eliminates the need for those outlandish expensive man made machines that man has built along with the costly errors of life and death of the humans involved.

With all this above knowledge of one's ability to diagnose, prescribe and heal all forms of diseases and illnesses, the wonder of it is that medicine should constantly be attempting to build ever more complicated and expensive machines at sky rocketing costs that can in no way compete or compare with the perfection of God's creation in every individual.

Remember - no man-made products, regardless of the cost, will ever successfully replace the perfection of God's creations.

The high rising costs of man-made products have risen beyond the ability of man to survive any good it may tend to serve such unnatural needs.

Medicine has reached a point where it has priced itself beyond the ability of man to buy it's offerings.

Nature has kept it's costs down to the normal level of supply and demand of simple fruits, herbs and other foods around the world.

Unscientific Medicine is always coming up with something new to prove it is a long way from meeting the needs of the people. But that something new, always means something more expensive, more complicated, more dangerous, more prone to side effects and farther and farther away from simple natural methods that are far less expensive and far more effective.

After all, if they would but study nature more closely and learn what God has to offer, they might just find the answers — the simple answers that have been there all the time — that really works and simply works fast.

Nature can be and is the best teacher after all. Surely nature knows far more than any and all of the Medical Profession, because God ordained it, regardless of how close to the Divine they may think they are.

Were it not better we reverse our present destructive course and give nature a chance to show what God can do? Let us do it now. Nature has been around a lot longer than any of the Medical doctors or their systems and will still be there long after man made plans fade away.

Returning to natural methods can reduce the need for most of the hospital care-less nursing care-less to no dangerous drugs and medication. Surgery can be almost a thing of the past, a horrible nightmare of faulty hopes of normal healing. Is this not what we need and are asking for? Just think of the misery and suffering and lives that can be saved by nature's methods. Are their lives not worth saving? Let nature prove it's methods work successfully since present medical methods are frought with a multitude of costly and deadly failures.

Medical Standards require nothing better — in spite of years of extensive and expensive research — than the practice of many addictive drugs and destructive surgery, until there is a cure. But if someone does come up with a cure for all diseases they will be treated — prosecuted — as a common criminal as treating is more lucrative than a cure.

Disease is Nature's imbalance asserting itself.
When one lives — so close — by or with — a faulty system — of errors — designed with only a part of the truth — one becomes blinded an dwary of change. Of such is our Medical system of Drugs a variety of injections and cutting ways.
The Medical system carries with it a deep responsibility and duties that requires more — much more — than ordinary mortals promote in resolving the true issues in fullness of the needs of the physical and spiritual balances in human exchanges of those who are sick Medicine lacks the knowledge to correct all diseases.

All the complete information on the Human Computer is given in my book intitled "Healing for the Age of Enlightenment"

FROM PAGE ONE

73,000 elderly die yearly from drug error, reaction, study says

By Nancy Weaver
Bee Staff Writer

Each year in this country, 73,000 elderly die from adverse drug reactions or medication errors.

In California, medication problems send an estimated 180,000 people to the hospital each year, and that health care costs the state more than $500 million, said Betty Yee of the State Senate Office of Research.

"Every year, more seniors die of medication, not of a disease but adverse medication reaction, than all the people who died in Vietnam," said Kathy Borgan, of the Chemical Dependency Center for Women in Sacramento.

Because the elderly take an estimated 30 percent of all prescribed drugs and 70 percent of all over-the-counter medications, they experience more problems with their usage, according to experts in elderly health care.

Often suffering from multiple health problems, an older person may be taking several medications prescribed by more than one doctor and may not be aware of how they conflict, said Borgan, who works with the senior medication education program.

Medications often have a stronger effect on an elderly person than on a younger patient and the prescribing doctor may not be aware of that difference, she said.

For example, some medications may linger in the body longer because the liver functions of an elderly person cannot work as quickly to process out the drugs, said Borgan, who speaks to senior citizens groups on drug usage.

The mixture of over-the-counter drugs can contribute to problems with a prescription. And, increasingly, older people are sharing pills, using outdated drugs or substituting medications because prescriptions are so expensive.

"Modern medicine makes it possible for the elderly to live richer lives than we ever imagined. But when medicines don't match what they need, then it becomes a menace," said Betty Brill, acting chairwoman of the Sacramento chapter of the California Medication Education Coalition.

Brill urges all patients to ask doctors to explain potential side effects or other warnings. Family members who notice a change in behavior or other possible effects of medication problems should consult a doctor.

Gardis Mundt, a member of Families of Overmedicated Elderly which is educating people about medication uses, said her mother was nearly fitted for a hearing aid until she discovered that her hearing loss was only a temporary side effect of her medication.

Her mother was waiting for Mundt to pick her up for her doctor's appointment when she read the fine print on the medication sample bottle given to her by her doctor. The sample bottle specified potential hearing loss as a side effect.

"She quit taking the medication and she didn't need the hearing aid," said Mundt. She said her mother's doctor hadn't cautioned her of the side effects.

The California Pharmacists Association is sponsoring a "brown bag" program for member pharmacists to screen an elderly person's prescriptions for problems such as dangerous drug interactions or outdated medications.

Elderly people are urged to throw all the drugs from their medicine cabinet into a brown paper bag and have them examined by a pharmacist participating in various screening programs being held at different times. For more information, call the association at 1-800-444-3851.

The use of sedatives and mind-altering medications by elderly people in their own homes also is a growing problem. Borgan said senior citizens in this country also take 40 percent of all prescribed antipsychotic or tranquilizing medications such as Valium, Haldol and Mellaril.

Borgan said such medications often help a person survive the loss of a spouse or friends but that they must be used with caution.

"That generation has that magic pill formula. They're ready to take medications, too eager to take them," said Morgan. "Part of the problem is that they're kind on innocent in some cases. They're being poisoned."

Notes

Notes

Notes

Notes

Notes

Notes